THE *Judy* & THE *Joy* OF

PASTA

SAUCES & SWEETS

THE *Judy* & THE *Joy* OF

PASTA

SAUCES & SWEETS

BY JUDY VIG AND JOY PAOLETTI

THE JUDY AND THE JOY OF PASTA SAUCES & SWEETS IS PUBLISHED BY JUDY AND JOY LLC.

COVER PHOTOGRAPH BY JAMIE ARABOLOS

FAMILY PHOTOGRAPHS COURTESY JUDY VIG & JOY PAOLETTI

PHOTOGRAPHS BY JOSEPH LAMBERT IMAGES

PHOTOGRAPH ON PG: II JAMIE ARABOLOS

PHOTOGRAPH ON PGS: X-XI BY VEER

PHOTOGRAPHS ON PGS: XII-1, 2-3, 21, 23, 24-25, 33, 39 AND 43 BY I-STOCK

PHOTOGRAPHS ON PGS: VIII, 50-51 AND 96 COURTESY OLD WORLD OLIVE CO.

COVER AND BOOK DESIGN BY KIRSTEN NAVIN

ISBN – 978-0-9910402-2-3

PRINTED IN THE UNITED STATES.

Our wonderful
and loving family

To our husbands: Chris and Jim, for all their patience
and support on this project and all the others, many thanks.

The Judy

Thank you to my children:

NICK: For your endless amount of patience and praise

JIMMY: For listening each and every time you called about my recipes when all you really wanted to know, "what's for dinner"

DANIELLE: Please stop asking me, "Mom did you sell any books yet? and when can we go shopping?"

The Joy

Thank you to my children:

PAULETTE: Thank you for offering to help with anything we asked!

CRISTYN: For printing the book text over and over again even though you kept saying, "Mom, just read it on the computer!"

PAIGE: For all the creative word suggestions you helped with when my old tired brain couldn't think anymore!

CAYLA: For being patient when I forgot each and every day everything you needed me to do that day!

Special thanks to our baby sister, Jackie, for taking over
all the family gatherings as we were writing this book.

And to our Mom, the best Mom in the whole world, for endless
phone calls explaining the family memories behind the recipes.

GROWING UP IN AN ITALIAN HOUSEHOLD, our family time was centered around the dinner table. Dad went to work while mom stayed home; so dinner time became the best part of the day, because that was when we were all together.

Mom cooked every night (move over June Cleaver!) and insisted on a well-balanced meal: which meant a protein, two vegetables and a starch were routinely on our plates. Something delicious was always on the stove bubbling away in the biggest pot. We would talk about what happened that day, cheerleading and what we were planning to wear the next day to school. Poor dad, how bored he must have been! Dad had five sisters so he was truly out numbered from birth; but what a life it was, full of food, fun and family.

We are busy moms, just like most of you, and have been juggling family, home and our work as television lifestyle chefs and food writers for many years. Don't be fooled by the fact that you can't tell us apart, we are identical twins but with completely opposite approaches to just about everything we do. *The Judy and the Joy of Pasta Sauces & Sweets* will bring you two perspectives on classic dishes.

THE JUDY: The shortcut, designed to help you to accomplish anything when time is at a minimum. *I take you from A-to-Z, in and out of the kitchen—fast, but without sacrificing presentation. "I don't want it fine, I want it fabulous!"*

THE JOY: The traditional way, for when you are able to plan ahead and let it simmer all day long. *I take you on a journey back in time to my grandmother's kitchen. Perfect for when there is plenty of time, money is no object, and the sky's the limit. For those with a love of detail, dedication and craftsmanship—this is the approach for you.*

A NOTE FROM JUDY:

"Joy thinks her traditional way of life is best, and frankly, I don't. I prefer to take the shortest, and quickest way possible and I'm always right."

A NOTE FROM JOY:

"Judy is wrong!"

It is with the long-time support and guidance of our parents and grandparents that we have pursued our love of cooking. With one sister, and seven children between us, we have cooked, baked, ached and faced every imaginable hurdle when it comes to: dinners, parties, lunches, brunches, and everything from sweet 16s to elegant bridal showers. Now in *The Judy and the Joy of Pasta Sauces & Sweets*, we give it to you straight—just in two different ways. Try them both and see which suits your personal style, perhaps even a combination of both.

We "Twin"cerely wish you The Judy and The Joy of life!

If it were not for the countless people and professionals we have met along the way who have extended: hours of their time, expertise, baking assistance, discounts on services (that were truly above and beyond), innumerable connections that opened doors, friendship, love, advice and a continued belief in us (and what we do), we would not be where we are today. We are eternally grateful to all of you.

To our Hersam Acorn Newspaper friends: for their patience regarding our column, which never meets its deadline on time!

ModernMom.com: for loving each and every recipe we send to the magazine

To our Better CT family: Scot Haney, Kara Sundlun, executive producer Jamie Mascia, Melissa Cole, everyone behind the camera and on set who have always been there for us, and lastly the security guard, who diligently puts up with us, every week, as we bang on the door until he lets us.in!

Frederick Paoletti Jr., we thank you for your time and unlimited patience when you had to repeat and explain the same thing to us countless times

Joe Lambert	*Lucinda Beatty aka "The Wig Lady"*
Jimmy the Baker	*David Kalman*
David Oralevich	*Becca Fera*
MaryJo Duffy	*John Krekoska*
Lisa Moyles	*Kirsten Navin*
Sue Bolen	*Marcy Ricardi*

CONTENTS

CONTENTS

BAKING:

Brownies

Coffee Cake

Chocolate Chip Cookies

Apple Crumble

BEAUTY:

HEALTH:

Rigatoni

Linguine
al Nero

Farfalle
Tricolore

Pappardelle

Ruote

Pasta Shapes

Eliche
Tricolori

Lumache

Linguine

- Thin, delicate pastas, like angel hair or thin spaghetti, are better served with light, thin sauces.
- Thicker pasta shapes, like fettuccine, work well with heavier sauces.
- Pasta shapes with holes or ridges, like mostaccioli or radiatore, are perfect for chunkier sauces.

· x ·

Tarfalle

Linguine
Pomodoro

Creste di Galli

Penne Tricolori

Tagliolini

Conchiglie

Conchiglioni Verdi
+ Pomorodoro

Chifferini

Tusilli Lunghi

There are almost
as many different pasta
shapes as we have cousins,
don't hesitate trying new
shapes. Just watch those
cooking times. If the pasta
fits...enjoy it!

Judy and Joy say:

· xi ·

Herbs

BASIL: One of the most popular herbs used in Italian cuisine. It's a necessity for pesto, and it pairs beautifully with tomatoes—the sweetness of the basil balances nicely with the acidity of the tomatoes.

BAY LEAF: Mostly used in soups and stews, make sure to remove the leaves before serving.

MARJORAM: Closely related to Oregano (and can be used as an alternative), however it's flavor is milder and more delicate.

MINT: There are hundreds of varieties of mint. These herbs run the gamut from mild and sweet to spicy and hot. Mint brings a unique freshness to recipes.

OREGANO: Marjoram's wild and more pungent, cousin. An essential ingredient in pizza sauce.

PARSLEY: Many people think of parsley as just a garnish; however, it is widely used in Italian cooking—especially the flat-leaf variety. Note: chewing on fresh parsley will eliminate the smell of garlic from your breath.

ROSEMARY: It's scent has been described as a combination of pine and mint. Rosemary is one of the strongest herbs, so use sparingly, a natural complement to potatoes, chicken, lamb, and beef.

SAGE: Is especially popular in Tuscany. A savory herb, frequently used in butter sauces.

THYME: The small thyme leaves pack a surprising punch; excellent for recipes where an earthy flavor is desired.

Red Sauces

Spaghetti & Meatballs

THE JUDY

Spaghetti & meatballs is one of my favorite Italian dishes. In our house it was always served on Sunday. One side of the family called it pasta and sauce, while the other side called it macaroni and gravy. Whatever you call it, it's full of white flour and way too many carbohydrates, add to that the calorie-laden meatballs and you have a very heavy meal. I love my healthier, lighter version of this classic that can be eaten anytime—not just for Sunday dinner—even twice a week.

For the sauce (or gravy), I love to use fresh ripe tomatoes. My choice for pasta is usually whole wheat; it's full of fiber with tons of vitamins and nutrients. I also select a very lean beef for the meatballs and mix-in healthier whole wheat bread crumbs rather than white.

Mangia!

JUDY'S HEALTHIER-SHORTER RECIPE

5	pounds of plum tomatoes
¼	cup olive oil
4-5	cloves of garlic, chopped
¼	cup fresh parsley, chopped

1	teaspoon fresh basil, chopped
	salt and pepper to taste
	a sprinkling of grated Parmesan cheese

Rinse tomatoes, core and cut in half. Place in a blender, or food processor, and puree until smooth. Set aside.

In a large heated saucepan add the garlic and sauté until golden. Add the tomatoes and remaining ingredients simmer for one hour.

MEATBALLS

¼	cup of cooked brown rice
¼	cup whole wheat bread crumbs
2	large eggs, lightly beaten
3	tablespoons milk
2	cloves garlic, minced

¾	cup grated Parmesan cheese
¼	cup chopped flat-leaf parsley
	salt and freshly ground black pepper
1	pound ground beef (90 percent lean or a ground sirloin)

Mix all of the ingredients together and shape into balls. Drop meatballs into simmering tomato sauce and let cook for about 45 minutes.

HEALTY TIPS & SUBSTITUTIONS

Everyone loves fresh herbs, but not everyone has access to an herb garden, especially year round. The solution: substitute oil and fresh garlic with the same proportion of a garlic infused olive oil. Experiment with flavors such as: Basil, Cilantro, or Sage. Herb olive oils become an herb garden at your fingertips.

Spaghetti & Meatballs

THE JOY

There is nothing better than the time-honored way to prepare spaghetti & meatballs. I remember Nana and Papa coming to visit from West Hartford to spend weekends with us. Papa was always carrying a big silver pot filled with Nana's heavenly red sauce, chock-full of the best meatballs ever! Every time I serve this family favorite, I giggle to myself at the memory of Papa coming in the front door of our childhood home carrying the Sunday sauce with the 'Italian elbow'!

Bon appetite Papa!

P.S. *'Italian elbow' refers to ringing the doorbell with your bent arm because your hands are busy carrying a pot filled with something delicious!*

TOMATO SAUCE

½ cup extra virgin olive oil	1½ - 2 cans of water (use cans from tomatoes)
2 large onions, finely chopped	½ glass red wine (more if you like)
4 cloves garlic, finely chopped	basil, chopped, optional
2 32 ounce cans crushed tomatoes	½ cup Parmesan cheese
1 32 ounce can tomato sauce	salt and black pepper to taste
2 tablespoons tomato paste	garlic and onion powder*

Sauté onions in ½ cup of oil for about 5 minutes, add the garlic and cook 1 minute more. Do not burn the garlic, it will become bitter. Add the 2 cans of crushed tomatoes, 1 can tomato sauce, and 2 tablespoons tomato paste. Let cook about 15 minutes and stir. Add water and stir until sauce comes to a medium boil. Add the wine, grated cheese and basil (if using). Stir then lower heat and allow to a simmer for about 2 hours. Taste and re-season adding garlic and onion powder* and enjoy!

*Mom adds a sprinkle of garlic and onion powder at the end. Stir and continue simmering.

"The tomato paste will help the sauce stick to the pasta". My mother must have said this 10 times to me on the day we were reviewing this recipe...I got it Mom...add the tomato paste!!

JOY'S TRADITIONAL MEATBALLS

½ cup plain bread crumbs	2 garlic cloves, minced
¼ cup flat-leaf parsley, chopped	½ teaspoon salt
2 large eggs, lightly beaten	¾ teaspoon freshly ground black pepper
2 tablespoons whole milk	1½ pound ground beef
¾ cup grated romano or Parmesan cheese	

Mix all the ingredients together and roll into balls any size you like! Drop meatballs into the simmering sauce for at least 1 hour.

Before rolling all of the meatballs, Nana would make a very tiny meatball the size of a quarter and drop it into the sauce, let it cook about 15 minutes then taste it. She did this so she could add more of anything if she needed to!

DID YOU KNOW?

There are a lot of opinions out there as to who created the popular dish, Spaghetti & Meatballs. We are going with Italian immigrants in the very early 20th century in New York City. They were the first to make it and the National Pasta Organization, which was originally named the National Macaroni Manufacturers Association, was the first organization to publish a recipe. Who knew?

A great way to get your family accustomed to whole-wheat pasta is to mix whole-wheat and white flour pasta together and ease into it. Soon they won't even notice!

GLUTEN FREE SUGGESTION use cornmeal, hominy grits or gluten free bread to replace traditional breadcrumbs. For the Pasta use your favorite gluten free pasta with ribbons of zucchini.

Mom always said if the sauce is bitter, add a whole carrot or two and let it cook in the sauce. A pinch of sugar is a favorite trick of Nana's too!

Joy's Tips & Tricks

Penne alla Vodka

THE JUDY

This is a great dish, but ohhhh...so fattening. I have tried over, and over, to make this dish using less butter, a fat-free cream and just a sprinkle of Parmesan cheese. It didn't work. To me, it's just not worth it. I feel, if you are going to eat Penne alla Vodka, then go ahead and enjoy it, just start your diet the next day. However, being forced to make it less hard on the thighs and belly for the sake of this book, I did play around with the recipe. I experimented, changing this, trying that, all to get rid of some of the fat and calories. After days of testing recipes it happened! I came up with a cold penne pasta salad with a bacon vodka dressing. Just remember, this recipe is for adults only.

COLD PENNE PASTA SALAD WITH A BACON VODKA VINAIGRETTE ALLA TINI

  8 ounces penne pasta, cooked
½ cup small grape tomatoes
¼ cup shallots
    shaved Parmesan cheese

THE VINAIGRETTE

3 tablespoons minced shallots
3 tablespoons red wine vinegar
3 tablespoons bacon vodka or to taste
3 tablespoons extra virgin olive oil

2 tablespoons honey
½ teaspoon salt
¼ teaspoon freshly ground black pepper

In a bowl, whisk together the shallots, red wine vinegar, bacon vodka, olive oil, honey, salt and black pepper. Toss with cooked pasta and the remaining ingredients.

Try using whole-wheat or gluten free pasta.

DID YOU KNOW?
Vodka adds a unique flavor when cooked with tomatoes. Some people say it adds a peppery flavor or a hint of citrus.

Penne alla Vodka

THE JOY

What can I say? This is the ultimate comfort food...fabulous and fattening. And with the edition of the salty bacon, I'm in heaven.

JOY'S PENNE ALLA VODKA RECIPE

1 tablespoon olive oil, once around the pan in a slow stream

2 tablespoons butter, or substitute a natural butter flavored oil

3 cloves garlic, minced

3 shallots, minced

½ cup vodka

1 cup chicken stock

1 32 ounce can crushed tomatoes

salt and fresh ground pepper

16 ounces pasta, such as penne or penne rigatte

½ cup heavy cream

Heat a large skillet over moderate heat. Add the oil, butter, and shallots. Gently sauté the shallots for three to five minutes to develop their sweetness. Add the garlic and cook for 1 minute. Pour the vodka into pan and reduce by half: 2-3 minutes. Add the chicken stock and tomatoes. Bring sauce to a slow bubble and reduce heat to simmer. Season with salt and pepper.

While the sauce is simmering away, cook your pasta of choice until al dente. Drain.

Stir cream into sauce. When the sauce returns to a small bubble, remove from heat. Toss the hot pasta with sauce.

DID YOU KNOW?
Along with people disco dancing at chic supper clubs in the mid 1970s, the very trendy Penne alla Vodka also came into fashion. And it continues to be one of the most popular dishes today.

HEALTY TIPS & SUBSTITUTIONS

There is a healthier option for butter—a dairy-free, butter flavored olive oil is the perfect substitute. Here are four prominent benefits:

1. It tastes just like butter, but has no dairy. Still 120 calories, but mono-saturated calories–healthy fat!
2. Natural Butter Oil is gluten free, vegan and 100% organic.
3. You use a lesser amount. For every 1 cup of butter, substitute only ¾ cup of butter olive oil.
4. Plus, it has a high smoke point–400 degrees.

My girls are always watching their weight, because of this I have switched from using heavy cream to fat-free half & half. It tastes fabulous and works beautifully in this recipe!

Joy's Tips & Tricks

Bolognese Sauce

THE JUDY

I adore classic Bolognese sauce...it is probably one of my favorites. I really love when Joy makes her sauce with beef, pork, veal and heavy cream—yes I said heavy cream! When it simmers on low for hours at a time, the entire house fills with the comforting aroma of...well, our Nana. Bolognese is a chunky, hearty, heavy sauce, full of calories and fat. And certainly not something you can make and serve in 30 minutes. It needs time, it has to simmer; so I am lightening it up and making it healthier. Plus it will be ready in a snap!

The most dramatic modification I made was to replace the meats with a bean. I love this, and I know you will too. I chose red kidney beans because they are high in fiber, low in fat (a lot lower), and they add a wonderful creaminess to the dish.

RED BEAN BOLOGNESE

1	14-ounce can red kidney beans, or other beans, rinsed and drained
2	tablespoons olive oil
1	small onion, chopped
½	cup chopped carrot
¼	cup chopped celery
	salt to taste

4	cloves garlic, chopped
½	cup white or red wine (whichever one you prefer)
1	14 ounce can diced tomatoes
¼	cup chopped fresh parsley, divided
8	ounces whole-wheat fettuccine
½	cup freshly grated Parmesan cheese

Prepare the whole wheat fettucini according to package directions, set aside.

Heat the oil in a medium saucepan over medium heat. Add the onion, carrot, celery and a sprinkling of salt and cook until softened: 10 minutes. Add the garlic cook 1 minute. Add the wine, increase heat to medium high and boil until most of the liquid evaporates: 3-4 minutes. Add the diced tomatoes, 2 tablespoons parsley and kidney beans. Bring to a low simmer for 15 minutes. Spoon into a food processor and whirl until the mixture is somewhat smooth, more like a sauce.

For a fabulous presentation, I decided to roast a tomato and scoop out the insides. I drizzled the tomato with olive oil and broiled it until the skin blistered. Be careful, you must watch it; or the tomato will burn. Mix the pasta and sauce together before filling.

HEALTY TIPS & SUBSTITUTIONS

Tuscan Herb olive oil is an Italian must for any pasta recipe. It substitutes well for other plain olive oils and is perfect for bread dipping.

Or try drizzling balsamic vinegar for a finishing, crowd-pleasing touch!

Bolognese Sauce

THE JOY

I have a large family; including four daughters with tons of friends, who are always at my house. They like to eat before cheerleading practice and after, before work and after...so pretty much all the time. I love to serve this recipe because once it is cooked; I can just leave it on the stove all day. The kids can then boil up fresh pasta anytime and just top it with the sauce.

JOY'S TRADITIONAL RECIPE

¼	pound pancetta, diced
1	medium size onion, diced
1	medium carrot, peeled diced
1	medium rib celery, diced
4	garlic cloves, minced
2	tablespoons olive Oil
½	pound ground sirloin
½	pound ground veal
½	pound ground pork

½ to 1	teaspoon sea salt (I like fine sea salt, but any is fine)
¼	teaspoon freshly ground black pepper
1	32 ounce can crushed tomatoes
½	glass dry red wine
½	cup milk or cream (I use fat-free half & half and it works fine)
	grated cheese for sprinkling

Heat the olive oil in large sauce pot. Cook the pancetta and minced vegetables on low heat, uncovered for about 30 minutes. Give it a stir every now and then. Add the ground meats, salt, pepper, and brown them up. Add the can of tomatoes and wine and simmer uncovered for about 45 minutes. Add the milk, or cream, a little at a time and stir.

Take a sip of wine, the kids will be home from school soon...with all of their friends.

Instead of
chopping the celery,
carrots and onions,
a quick whirl in the food
processor has the
job done
in seconds!

Joy's Tips & Tricks

Lasagna

THE JUDY

Lasagna soup was a huge hit with my family, the only complaint was that there wasn't enough for leftovers. I broke the lasagna noodles into big chunks. They have a perfect chewy texture (al dente of course), and swimming in a rich tomato broth; it was sheer bliss. I topped the soup with a scoop of creamy Parmesan ricotta in the center—it took my breath away. So simple, and so fast to make; who the heck wants to make it the traditional way? NOT ME!

LASAGNA SOUP

2 -3	tablespoons olive oil
1	pound ground Italian sausage
1	onion, diced
2	cloves garlic, chopped
2	pounds fresh tomatoes (I used campari tomatoes)
2	tablespoons tomato paste

4	cups chicken broth (I used store bought)
	salt and pepper to taste
¼-½	cups grated Parmesan cheese
½	cup red wine
½	pound lasagna noodles broken into large pieces

Heat the oil in a large soup pot. Add the sausage and cook until browned. Add the onions and garlic cook for another 3-4 minutes. Add the tomatoes, chicken broth, tomato paste, wine and Parmesan cheese. Let simmer for an hour, taste and re-season.

About 10 minutes before you are ready to serve add the torn lasagna noodles to the soup pot. They may take a bit longer to cook, so keep checking. More broth may need to be added at this point to compensate for the large chunks of noodles. I also brought another pot of salted water to a boil in order to cook some additional noodles.

Ladle the soup into big bowls and top with a dollop of ricotta right in the center! Crusty bread is the perfect accompaniment.

Any shape pasta will work perfectly in this dish.

PARMESAN RICOTTA

4	ounces ricotta
¼	cup Parmesan, grated
¼	mozzarella, shredded

1	tablespoon basil and parsley, chopped
	salt and pepper to taste

Mix all the ingredients together (except for the salt and pepper), check for saltiness before adding any salt, the Parmesan cheese is salty on its own. Season with pepper

GLUTEN FREE SUGGESTION
Gluten free lasagna noodles and brown rice noodles are available; if not in your supermarket, try a speciality food store. An even healthier choice would be to replace the noodles with slices of zucchini or eggplant, or try a combination of both!

DID YOU KNOW?

The time consuming task of boiling noodles used to be a requirement for lasagna but now no-boil noodles exist!

Lasagna can be made in the dishwasher, are you serious? Yes!!! Prepare your lasagna as normal using whichever noodle you choose (boil or no boil) and cover tightly with aluminum foil. Use the heated dry and sanitize cycle on your dishwasher to cook the lasagna.

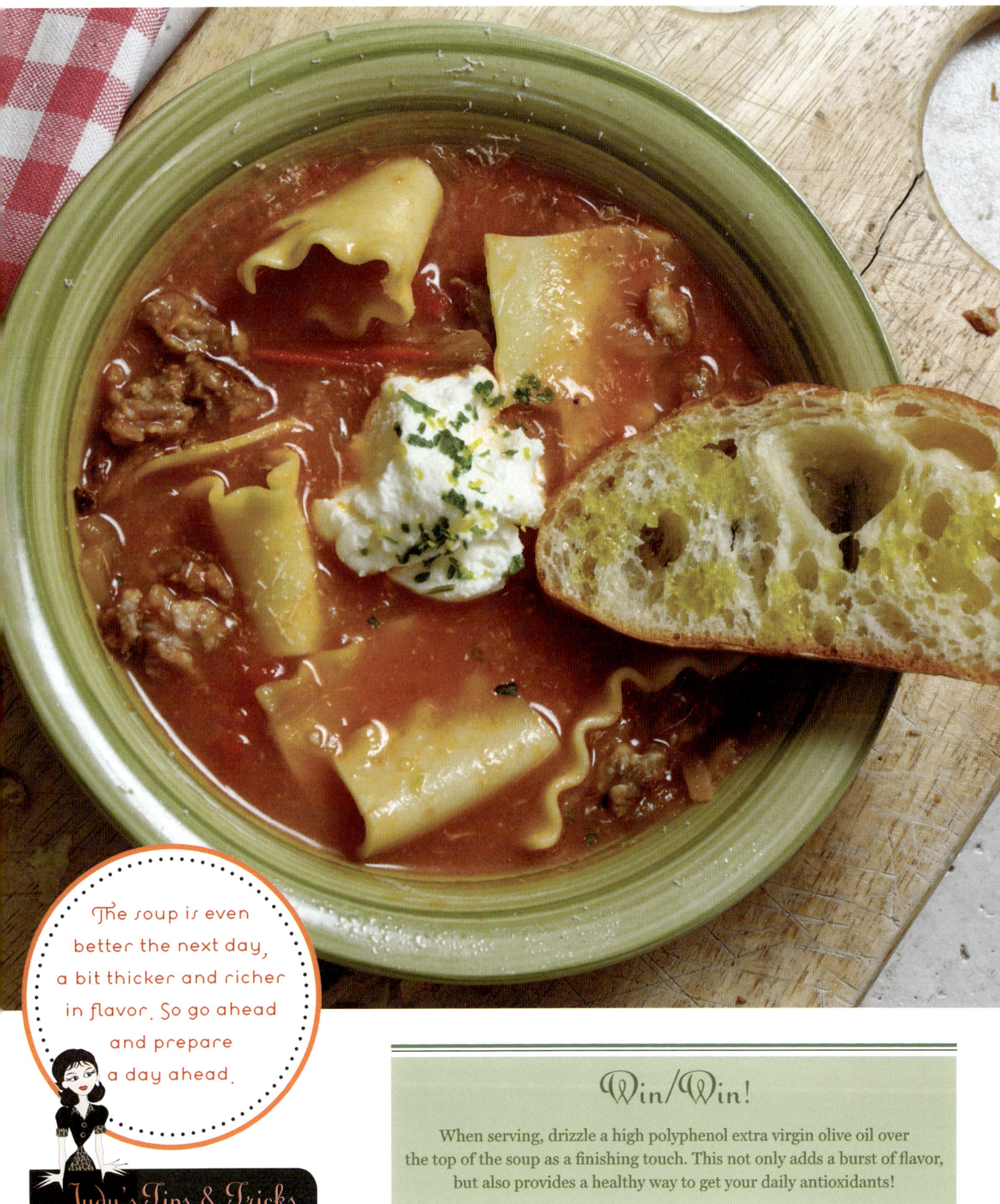

The soup is even better the next day, a bit thicker and richer in flavor. So go ahead and prepare a day ahead.

Judy's Tips & Tricks

Win/Win!

When serving, drizzle a high polyphenol extra virgin olive oil over the top of the soup as a finishing touch. This not only adds a burst of flavor, but also provides a healthy way to get your daily antioxidants!

Lasagna

THE JOY

Today there are so many different ways to prepare lasagna. It can be made using your favorite meat such as: beef, turkey, chicken, pork, 'saus-a-veech' (that's how we say sausage!), it can even be vegetarian, using fresh vegetables along with a variety cheeses. The sky is the limit when it comes to this amazing dish, so be creative and have fun!

TRADITIONAL LASAGNA RECIPE

Your family sauce recipe
(mine has ground sausage this time)

3   pounds fresh ricotta cheese

3   large egg yolks

1   cup grated Parmesan cheese

Salt to taste

¼   teaspoon fresh ground black pepper

handful of chopped parsley

1   pound no cook lasagna noodles, or regular boiled noodles if you prefer

1   pound fresh shredded mozzarella cheese

Preheat oven to 400 degrees and butter an 11 x 14 x 3-inch baking pan.

Bring sauce to room temperature.

In a large bowl, mix together the ricotta cheese, egg yolks and Parmesan cheese. Stop and taste before you add any salt. Add black pepper and parsley.

Spread about 3 cups of the sauce on the bottom of the prepared baking dish. Place a layer of noodles on top of the sauce, overlap a bit if you wish. Spread about 2 cups of the sauce over the noodles and half of the ricotta mixture on top of the sauce. Top with another layer of lasagna noodles.

Repeat with more sauce and the remaining ricotta mixture. Top with a final layer of lasagna noodles and finish with a layer of shredded mozzarella.

Bake until the sauce is bubbling and the cheese is melted, at least 1 hour. If the cheese starts to brown, cover with aluminum foil. Let the lasagna stand 10-15 minutes before serving.

Sauce can be prepared a day ahead of time.

Earthy Goodness

A fun twist on this favorite is to drizzle a porcini flavored olive oil over the top, it gives the dish a rich flavorful bite.

DID YOU KNOW?
Originally, the word "lasagna" did not refer to the food, instead "lasagna" denoted the dish it was cooked in. The earliest lasagna recipes date back to the thirteenth century. Europeans were not familiar with tomatoes at that time, and so tomatoes were not even used in initial versions of lasagna.

Cover unbaked, and refrigerate up to one day in advance, or freeze, unbaked, up to three weeks in advance. Defrost overnight in the refrigerator; bake as directed.

To check if the lasagna is hot through out, Mom would stick a butter knife carefully into the middle and hold it there for a few seconds. If the knife is hot to the touch when you pull it out, it is ready to go!

Joy's Tips & Tricks

Pasta Puttanesca

Chickpeas (garbanzo beans) are a perfect match for this thick Italian red sauce. Actually, I prefer my puttanesca with chickpeas, rather than on pasta, and I feel better after eating it. It's a wonderful alternative if you are sensitive to gluten.

JUDY'S PUTTANESCA WITH CHICK PEAS

1	pound fresh tomatoes, diced
8	anchovy fillets, minced
1/2	cup pitted Kalamata olives, coarsely chopped
3	tablespoons capers, rinsed
1/4	cup parsley, finely chopped

3-4	cloves garlic, minced or pressed
2-3	tablespoons extra virgin olive oil
1	teaspoon red chili flakes
2	cups canned chickpeas

Press or finely mince the garlic. Heat a large pan on medium and add 2 tablespoons olive oil. When the olive oil swirls easily in the pan add the anchovies, garlic mixture and chili flakes. Stir continuously until garlic just begins to brown, about 2 minutes, add the tomatoes and simmer.

Allow tomatoes to cook, stirring occasionally. If the tomatoes begin to stick to the bottom of the pan, add 1/4 cup water to thin the sauce. You may need to do this several times depending upon the variety of tomato. When the tomatoes begin to soften, use a wooden spoon to crush them a bit in the pan to create smaller chunks.

After the sauce has simmered about 12-15 minutes toss in the capers, olives, and parsley. Mix to combine. I toss in some excellent olive oil at this point to brighten it up.

Pepper is a nice addition, but salt is probably not necessary because of the anchovies.

To save time, use a chopped tomato in the box.

GLUTEN FREE SUGGESTION

It already is! but go ahead and throw in some gluten free pasta if you like!

Judy's Tips & Tricks

Pasta Puttanesca

DID YOU KNOW?

There are three very funny Italian tales about this hot and spicy sauce.

1. Bordello ladies preferred this easy sauce because it could be made quickly between servicing customers.

2. Wives would throw leftovers of the pasta dish while screaming, Puttana, Puttana! at the above mentioned ladies as they walked by.

3. The sauce was a favorite of married women who wanted to spend less time in the kitchen; and more time with their husbands in the bedroom!

THE JOY

The traditional pasta paired with this recipe is spaghetti, but any pasta your family prefers is just fine! We have used all types: penne, buccatini (Judy's favorite) and linguini. The dish is tangy and a bit salty from the capers; as for spice, you can make it as hot as you like. When we were teens, every time our mom served this dish for dinner, she would tell us a silly story that long ago the ladies of the evening would place pots of puttanesca in their windows to tempt men into their bordellos. We would laugh trying to picture this story in our minds as we shoveled forkfuls of the delicious spaghetti into our mouths.

JOYS TRADITIONAL RECIPE

¼ cup olive oil	2 tablespoons drained capers
1 cup finely chopped onion	2 tablespoons minced anchovy fillets (about 8 fillets)
6 cloves minced garlic	½ teaspoon dried crushed basil
2 28 ounce cans Roma plum tomatoes, crushed with juice	½ teaspoon dried crushed red pepper flakes
1 cup tightly packed, pitted, and halved Kalamata olives	Salt, optional (taste first)
2 tablespoons tomato paste	1 pound penne pasta, cooked al dente

In a large pot heat the olive oil over medium high heat. Add the onion and sauté until soft and lightly caramelized, about 6 minutes. Add the garlic and cook an additional 2 minutes. Add the tomatoes and the remaining ingredients and simmer until the sauce has thickened and is slightly reduced: 40 minutes. Adjust seasoning to taste, cover and set aside. Add the spaghetti to the pan and stir.

Taste sauce before adding salt. The capers, olives and the anchovies tend to be salty on their own.

Joy's Tips & Tricks

Cream Sauces

Fettuccine Alfredo

THE JUDY

Thank God there is a lighter, healthier approach for this fabulous dish! The yogurt blended with the ricotta cheese makes a wonderful, light sauce; mild in flavor, completely satisfying, and totally guilt free! I like to use Greek yogurt rather than regular because it has a thicker, creamier texture and is higher in protein than most other yogurts. I am so happy about this dish; I love to lighten up my recipes for my body, and this one feeds my soul too!

JUDY'S HEALTHY VERSION FETTUCCINE ALFREDO

8 ounces angel hair pasta

1 tablespoon or more of olive oil, or try a natural butter olive oil

1 shallot, sliced

1 garlic clove minced (some times I sprinkle on garlic powder instead, 1/4 teaspoon)

1 cup low-fat plain Greek yogurt

1 cup low-fat ricotta cheese

1/2 cup Parmesan cheese

1/2 teaspoon lemon zest, optional

kosher salt to taste, check sauce first before adding

freshly ground black pepper

reserved pasta water

Boil and cook the pasta according to package directions. Drain well, reserving about 1 cup of the pasta water.

In a large skillet on medium high heat add the olive oil and sauté shallots until soft. Add the garlic and cook a few minutes longer. Lower the heat to medium low and add the yogurt, low-fat ricotta, Parmesan cheese and lemon zest (if you are using it). Stir with a wooden spoon. If the sauce is too thick, add the pasta water one spoonful at a time.* Continue to stir and add more water until desired consistency is reached. Add the pasta to sauce pan and toss to coat, serve immediately.

This is a great technique to thin the sauce to your preferred texture.

 For a quick protein boost add shrimp or chicken.

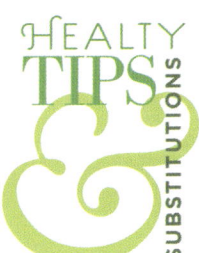

Replace the pasta entirely by using ribbons of zucchini squash to cut even more carbs and calories.

Judy's Tips & Tricks

HEALTY TIPS & SUBSTITUTIONS

Too add a boost of lemon flavor, try a lemon olive oil with the zest of fresh lemons. Great for when you don't have any lemons in the house.

For even more lemony goodness, use a lemon balsamic vinegar for a burst of citrus flavor. Don't be afraid to experiment, vinegar has only 10 calories per tablespoon. It tastes great and balsamics aid in digestion.

Fettuccine Alfredo

THE JOY

There is something about a bowl of creamy Fettuccine Alfredo that makes my mouth water. In this recipe the cream, butter, cheeses, and subtle flavor of garlic make a delightful sauce that perfectly coats the pasta. I love the way the pasta slips through my lips surrounded by the velvety sauce. Yum! This isn't a light dish, and certainly not the healthiest, but you need to spoil yourself every now and then. Judy likes to remind me that every once in a while a little indulgence is good for your spirit.

FETTUCCINE ALFREDO

- 1 pound fettuccine noodles cooked and drained, reserve some of the pasta water
- 1 stick butter or substitute with 6 tablespoons natural butter oil
- 3 garlic cloves, sliced

- 1 cup heavy cream
- salt and pepper, to taste
- 1½ cups freshly grated Parmesan cheese, start with this you can add more if you like

Cook pasta according to package directions.

In a warm saucepan or skillet, melt the butter, add garlic and cook one minute. Add the cream and season with freshly ground black pepper. Sprinkle in half of the cheese and stir, check for saltiness before sprinkling on the salt. Add pasta, toss.

At this point you may need to add some of the reserved pasta water to thin the sauce. Add in the rest of the Parmesan cheese, toss quickly and serve immediately.

Gluten Free or brown rice pasta can be substituted

A Higher Plane

Fettuccini Alfredo is absolutely divine with a tablespoon or two of
white truffle oil stirred into the sauce
just before serving, or added individually to each plate.

A great way
to thin the sauce
is by adding a little
of the hot pasta
water to it.

Joy's Tips & Tricks

Lemon Cream Sauce

I love the freshness that lemons bring to any recipe. Our mom would say, "It just brightens it up a bit". And she is right. I often find myself saying, "What does this recipe need?" And the answer usually is "it needs a bit of citrus". While I was working on this healthier recipe for lemon cream sauce, I knew fresh lemon zest would help balance the twang of the yogurt. The result is a bright, fresh sauce.

PASTA WITH LEMON CREAM SAUCE

8	ounces pasta, whole wheat, gluten free or high-protein pasta
½	cup nonfat Greek yogurt
¼	cup grated Parmesan cheese
1-2	teaspoon(s) grated lemon zest
¼	teaspoon salt, taste first
¼	teaspoon cracked black pepper

1-2	tablespoon(s) extra virgin olive oil,
2	garlic cloves, minced
½	shallot, minced
2	tablespoons parsley, minced
2	tablespoons chives, minced

Boil pasta according to package directions and set aside, I used cavatappi for this presentation. Save ¼ cup pasta water.

In a skillet on medium heat, sauté shallots and garlic in olive oil until soft: 3-4 minutes. Add the yogurt, Parmesan, salt, pepper and lemon zest.

Add in the drained pasta. Stir to combine and add some of the reserved pasta water and taste it. Adjust any seasoning to your liking. A sprinkling of parsley and chives for the garnish, and you're good to go!

Use small pasta like tubetini or baby shells and serve cold. I love to present it in a hollowed out fresh lemon for either a luncheon or as an appetizer at my dinner parties!

Judy's Tips & Tricks

HEALTY TIPS & SUBSTITUTIONS

Who would resist a swapping butter for oil when it means less fat (also a healthier fat), and lower calories while keeping the same great taste! Natural butter flavored olive oil is at your service. For an authentic Italian lemon flavor try a Lemon flavored olive oil

Lemon Cream Sauce

THE JOY

This is a great spring dish, and a favorite of ours at Easter time. A few years ago when I was in Italy we had this dish at a local restaurant. The lemons were as big as oranges and much sweeter than we have here in the states. The lemon flavor adds a hint of brightness and makes the sauce so refreshing.

SPAGHETTI WITH LEMON CREAM SAUCE AND ASPARAGUS

1	pound asparagus	3	tablespoons butter or substitute
2	large shallots	2	tablespoons natural butter Olive Oil
2	lemons	3/4	cup heavy cream
1	pound dried spaghetti or fettuccine		

Trim the asparagus, cut on diagonal into 1/4-inch thick slices. Finely chop the shallots. Finely grate lemon zest to measure 1 1/2 teaspoons, and squeeze enough juice to measure 3 tablespoons.

Cook the asparagus in boiling water until tender and yet still crisp, about 3 minutes.
Drain and set aside.

In a deep 12-inch heavy skillet cook the shallots in butter on low heat: 5 minutes. Season with salt and pepper to taste. Stir in the cream and zest. Simmer, then add 2 tablespoons lemon juice. Take skillet off the heat.

Cook the pasta in boiling water until al dente in firmness. Reserve 1 cup pasta water. Drain pasta and add to sauce along with the asparagus, 1/2 cup pasta water, remaining tablespoon lemon juice, and salt and pepper to taste. Heat mixture over low heat and toss.

DID YOU KNOW?

Lemon Cream Sauce is extremely versatile. As a savory sauce, it's great when flavored with garlic, basil and Parmesan cheese served over pasta, chicken, veal or fish. But it's also a wonderful dessert sauce and can be used in cupcakes, puddings, as a cake filling, or even just on its own.

A fresh grating of lemon zest on top adds extra zing and looks fabulous. You can also decorate the plate with a lemon slice or an edible pansy...perfect for a spring meal!

Joy's Tips & Tricks

Pasta Carbonara

I love this recipe but don't understand why it couldn't be just as fabulous with healthier ingredients. All that fat from the cream and the bacon is a heart attack waiting to happen, and just not necessary. I always substitute heavy cream with a fat-free half & half or fat-free cream for my cream based sauces...my family never knows the difference! Replacing regular bacon with turkey bacon is a beneficial choice as well. It's delicious and has 50% less fat than regular bacon..

JUDY'S HEALTHY SPAGHETTI CARBONARA

8 ounces brown rice pasta	3 cloves garlic, minced
1 cup Egg Beaters®	½ cup parsley, chopped, saving some for garnish
½ cup shredded Parmesan cheese	1 teaspoon ground black pepper
splash of fat free heavy cream (optional, I love a splash or two of this)	salt to taste
1 tablespoon extra virgin olive oil	2 slices of turkey bacon cooked for crumbling on top, (½ slice of bacon for each, more if you want)
3 shallots, chopped	

Cook pasta in a large pot.

In a large skillet add the olive oil and sauté shallots until soft. Add the garlic and cook one more minute. Turn heat down to low.

In a separate bowl beat the Egg Beaters®, Parmesan cheese, parsley (about half) and cream (if using) add to skillet and stir until combined.

Drain the pasta and add to skillet. Toss quickly until egg mixture cooks.

Sprinkle with the turkey bacon crumbles.

The splash of fat-free cream adds creaminess to the dish with out all the calories. You can also use fat-free evaporated milk.

Use any pasta you like. Whole wheat or spinach would be delish. I like brown rice pasta a lot, it's light, and doesn't cause bloating the way regular pasta does.

Judy's Tips & Tricks

Pasta Carbonara

THE JOY

This recipe is truly my favorite. I know that I say that about all of my recipes, but this one is de-lush. There is just no other word. The eggy sauce clings to each strand of the spaghetti perfectly, and with a very generous helping of grated Parmesan cheese and heavy cream...this recipe goes right to ah-maz-ing!

PASTA CARBONARA

1	pound pasta, cooked al dente (any kind)
5	eggs
½	cup heavy cream
	salt and freshly ground black pepper to taste
1	tablespoon extra virgin olive oil

2	tablespoons butter or substitute with Old World Olive Co. Natural Butter olive oil
½	pound pancetta, bacon, prosciutto or salt pork,
3	garlic cloves
1¼	cups freshly grated Parmesan and/or romano cheese

Cut the pancetta, bacon, prosciutto or salt pork into small ⅛-inch cubes. Add the 3 whole, peeled garlic cloves.

In a large heavy skillet over low heat, sauté the meat bits and garlic for 10 minutes or so, until the meat becomes translucent and softened. Press the softened garlic into the oil from the bacon. Add additional olive oil as needed to keep bits from sticking.

Meanwhile, cook the pasta until al dente and drain

Beat the eggs and cream together. Add a pinch of salt.

Add butter to pan and stir until melted. Stir the cooked pasta into the skillet. Remove pan from heat and stir in the beaten egg/cream mixture along with half of the grated cheese. Stir quickly as the heat of the pasta will begin to cook the eggs. Stir until each strand of spaghetti is well coated. Toss in remaining cheese. Salt and pepper to taste. Serve at once.

DID YOU KNOW?

This Pasta dish originated in Rome and is said to be the favorite dish of the coal miners. Long ago the men would go out to the woods for months at a time. They packed most of the ingredients for this recipe and would look for fresh eggs at local farms they happened to come upon. The men would cook over an open flame in big cast iron pots, it was a quick and an easy meal for them to toss together at the end of a long day.

Serve a poached egg on top of each dish. This puts the presentation way over the top! You can use a raw egg on top if it is pasteurized and you feel safe doing so.

Joy's Tips & Tricks

Savory Ravioli

THE JUDY

For my healthier take on raviolis, instead of using a pasta dough, I am loving the ease of a wonton wrapper. They are commonly used for a chinese dumpling, but work great and are just as delicious! They are a bit lower in calories, and when filled with my scrumptious filling of butternut squash and carmelized onions they are just delightful! With a drizzle of a good quality olive oil which is full of antioxidents, you will be in for a treat!

BUTTERNUT SQUASH RAVOILI

1	large butternut squash, peeled and seeded and cut in 1-inch chunks
1	egg yolk
3	tablespoons olive oil
2	teaspoons sea salt

1	teaspoon onion powder
1	teaspoon freshly ground black pepper
	Wonton wrappers
	Olive Oil for drizzling

CARAMELIZED ONIONS

1	large sweet onion, minced
2-3	tablespoons olive oil
	pinch of salt and pepper

Heat sauté pan to medium heat. Swirl onion pieces in oil to coat. Let the onions cook slowly for about 30 minutes, or longer if necessary, until caramel in color. Set aside.

Preheat the oven to 400° F. Drizzle squash with the olive oil, salt, and pepper then toss well. Arrange the squash on a sheet pan in one layer and roast for 25-30 minutes, or until tender. Allow to cool. Mash the squash and add nutmeg, pinch of salt, pepper, onion powder and parmesan cheese and egg yolk, blend until smooth. Taste & re-season as desired.

Add caramelized onions to butternut mixture.

Lay wrappers, whichever you have chosen, on a parchment lined baking sheet. Fill wrappers with about a tablespoon of filling. Wet the rim of the pasta sheets with water. Lay another pasta sheet, or wonton wrapper, on top of the squash filling and seal the edges making sure not to trap air bubbles inside the ravioli. Bring a large pot of water to a boil. Add a tablespoon or two of salt to the water. Lower heat to a gentle boil and place the pasta into the pot. Raviolis are done when they float and are fully cooked. Remove with a slotted spoon.

Drizzle with a good quality olive oil and a sprinkle of freshly grated parmesan cheese.

DID YOU KNOW?
The ravioli is a popular Italian dish enjoyed by all| They are like little pillows, stuffed with all different types of fillings. Some are filled with savory ingredients and some sweet..yes a ravioli can be sweet| They can be boiled, baked, toasted or fried and tossed or topped with sauces or syrups.

To make this recipe a snap use canned squash and rice wrappers (also called rice papers and spring roll wrappers)

Joy's Tips & Tricks

Butter Sauce

THE JOY
Just a drizzle of a wonderfully flavored olive oil can dress up a simple meal and turn it into a great one. Below I used a three cheese ravioli, fried lightly in garlic butter, garnished with Parmesan and fresh parsley. Using a fragrant olive oil drizzle for the finish was just perfect!

THREE CHEESE RAVIOLI IN FRIED BUTTER SAUCE

1 pound ravioli, prepared according to package directions	parsley, minced for garnish
2 garlic cloves, minced	Parmesan cheese, garnish
2 -3 tablespoons butter	salt and pepper to taste
	olive oil for drizzle

Prepare ravioli according to package directions. Drain and lay on paper towels to blot excess water.

In a frying pan melt the butter and sauté garlic until soft. Add the ravioli in batches and fry on each side: 3-4 minutes, or until golden brown. Season with salt and pepper.

Transfer to a decorative plate and garnish with cheese and parsley. Before serving drizzle with a quality olive oil.

The ravioli can
be cooked a day ahead.
Store in a single layer
and keep refrigerated until
ready to fry and serve hot
to your guests.

Joy's Tips & Tricks

Wedding Bell Soup

THE JUDY

This soup was served on my wedding day as Mom requested. It was as beautiful sitting in a little china bowl as it was delicious. Although Joy's traditional recipe is pretty perfect, I wanted to change a few things to make it more nutritious, if thats even possible...but you know me! I am adding chopped celery, carrots and potato. Did I mention my version is meatless? Yes, meatless! You don't need to eat meat all the time. I am using quinoa and freshly grated parmesan cheese along with the rest of the ingredients. I think you will be pleasantly surprised.

JUDY'S MEATLESS WEDDING BELL SOUP

3-4 tablespoons good quality olive oil	8 cups of chicken broth, homemade or store bought
3 cloves of garlic, minced	1/4 cup parmesan cheese
3 carrots, chopped	meatless meatballs, recipe follows
2 celery stalks, chopped	
2 potatoes, chopped	

Just like in Joys directions we will use a 6 quart sauce pan and saute the garlic in the olive oil: 2-3 minutes. Add chopped carrots and celery, saute about one more minute. Add broth, potatoes, and grated cheese. Simple and delish!

MEATLESS MEATBALLS

1/3 cup bread crumbs	1/4 cup minced shallot
2/3 cups quinoa	2 large garlic cloves, minced
2 large eggs	Salt & Pepper to taste
1/2 cup coarsely grated carrot	1/4 cup olive oil
1/2 cup coarsely grated summer squash	
1/2 cup grated parmesan cheese, I like to mix parmesan and romano	

In a medium saucepan, cook the quinoa in boiling water until just tender, about 10 minutes. Drain and spread quinoa on a baking sheet to cool. In a bowl, whisk the eggs. Squeeze the liquid from the zucchini and carrots and add to the eggs. Stir in the cheese, shallot, garlic, salt and pepper. Mix in the quinoa and bread crumbs. Let stand for 10 minutes.

Use a 1/4-cup measure, roll into round balls and add to simmering soup and cook about 30 mins.

I love using this recipe and forming into patties and cooking in a bit of olive oil as a veggie-ish burger!

DID YOU KNOW?

That in Italian this soup is called Minestra Maritata which means "married soup"? Or that most people think that it is called Wedding Bell Soup because it is served at Italian weddings? That is simply not true! "Married soup" means the veggies and the meat come together perfectly like a good marriage.

I like to us store bought organic chicken broth in a box as opposed to most canned brands that have high levels of pba

Judy's Tips & Tricks

Wedding Bell Soup

THE JOY

This is a special dish in the Italian home. Our Great grandmother Nellie always made this soup, and our Nana has passed it on to us. For our family, this delicate soup was always served after the antipasto in Nana's beautiful china soup bowls that she received from her parents as a wedding gift. Truly heartwarming and delicious! Mom insisted that this be served at all of our weddings with a drizzle of olive oil floating gracefully on the top! It looks like a lot for this soup to come together, but it really is easy!

WEDDING BELL SOUP

2 cloves garlic, sliced	S'wepper to taste (salt with pepper), recipe follows*
3-4 tablespoons Old World Olive Co Extra Virgin Olive Oil	¼ cup Parmesan cheese
2 carrots, chopped very small	2 cups of cooked pasta, anything small, we like pastina
8 cups of chicken broth, (homemade or store bought)	
2 medium heads of escarole, cleaned and chopped	

In a 6-quart sauce pan, saute the garlic in olive oil: 2 -3 minutes. Add the chicken broth and bring to a boil for 5 minutes, reduce heat to medium.

Drop the meatballs (recipe follows) into the broth and add the chopped escarole. When the meatballs rise to the top they are just about done, but cook at least 20 minutes more in broth (double check to see if they are cooked through). Add the Parmesan cheese and taste before adding S'wepper (Parmesan cheese is salty) Add the 2 cups cooked macaroni, done! Enjoy!

MINI MEATBALLS

1 pound ground beef	1 teapoon S'wepper (salt with pepper), recipe follows*
½ cup plain bread crumbs	1 clove of garlic, very finely chopped
¼ cup chopped parsley	¼ teaspoon garlic powder (or to taste)
1 egg, lightly beaten	¼ teaspoon onion powder
½ cup grated parmesan cheese	

Mix all the ingredients together and roll into tiny meatballs. I used a well rounded tablespoon to measure these tiny gems!

*S'wepper: a mix of salt & pepper. Two parts salt to one part pepper. Mix, store and ready to go!

This soup can be prepared well ahead of time and frozen. Add your pasta before serving. Ugh...if you have too, you can use a prepared beef broth.

Joy's Tips & Tricks

· 45 ·

Tiramisu

THE JUDY

A fabulous dessert and a staple in our home, but packed with way too many calories! After a little thought and experimenting I came up with a lighter version that is still rich in flavor and completely satisfying. Our Aunt Lena used to make a meringue cookie, which we call "schoomie's". Please do not ask us why she chose this silly name—to this day no one knows! They were a crisp meringue flecked with sweet chocolate (always a favorite in our family). I decided to pipe the meringue into kiss shaped cookies and sandwich them with a more healthful filling rather than the traditional mascarpone. The result was bellisimo! Ciao!

COFFEE MERINGUES

4	egg whites (room temperature)	1	cup superfine sugar
¼	teaspoon cream of tartar	2½	teaspoons espresso powder

Preheat oven to 225°F.

Separate the eggs and bring to room temperature (save yolks for another use).

Mix the espresso powder with the superfine sugar.

Place room temperature egg whites in a metal or glass bowl. Begin beating the eggs until they start to thicken. Add the cream of tartar and continue beating eggs until soft peaks form.

Gradually begin to add the sugar to the egg whites. Do this SLOWLY and in a steady stream (while still beating). Continue beating the mixture until it is glossy and stiff peaks form (you'll need to beat the mixture on a high speed at this point). Unsure that the sugar is fully incorporated by running some of the meringue between two fingers, you should not feel any sugar grains.

Line your baking sheet with parchment paper. Spoon the meringue mixture into a piping bag with a large star tip (or like I do, spoon it into a plastic bag and snip the tip off).

Bake for two hours. DO NOT open the door during the baking process. Turn off the oven and let them stay inside the oven until the oven completely cools down.

RICOTTA CHEESE FILLING RECIPE

1	cup part skim ricotta cheese	1	teaspoon rum
2	tablespoons powdered sugar		mini chocolate chips or shavings can be added (optional)
2	teaspoons vanilla extract		

In a small bowl combine the ricotta cheese, powdered sugar, vanilla and rum. Stir thoroughly to combine all of the ingredients, cover and cool in the refrigerator.

ASSEMBLY

Put these together just before serving because the moisture will melt the meringue. Coat one of the meringue kisses on the flat side with ricotta cheese filling and sandwich with another meringue kiss.

Tiramisu

THE JOY

This is the most popular dessert for Italians. While many variations and presentations have evolved over the years, the one consistent ingredient has always been the mascarpone cheese. Traditional Tiramisu made in Italy contained raw eggs; today, because of the danger of salmonella contamination, we prefer to cook the yolks with the sugar in a double boiler to reduce any risk.

JOY'S TRADITIONAL TIRAMISU

6	egg yolks
3	tablespoons sugar
1	pound mascarpone cheese
1½	cups strong espresso, cooled

2	teaspoons dark rum
24	packaged ladyfingers
½	cup bittersweet chocolate shavings, for garnish

Combine the egg yolks and sugar in the top of a double boiler. Beat at medium speed with an electric mixer until thick and lemon-colored. Place over boiling water and reduce heat to medium-low, cook 10 minutes constantly stirring. Add the mascarpone cheese and beat until smooth. Add 1 tablespoon of espresso, mix thoroughly. In a small shallow dish add the remaining espresso and rum.

Dip each ladyfinger into the espresso and rum mixture for 5 seconds. If you let the ladyfingers soak too long, they will fall apart. Place the soaked ladyfingers on the bottom of a 13 x 9-inch baking dish, breaking them in half in order to entirely cover the bottom. Spread ½ of the mascarpone filling over the ladyfingers. Add another layer of soaked ladyfingers and top with remaining mascarpone mix.

Cover tiramisu with plastic wrap and refrigerate for at least 2 hours and up to 8 hours. Before serving sprinkle with chocolate shavings.

 Prepare some extra coffee just in case the quantity is not enough.

Any coffee flavored liqueur can be used; Kahlua®, Brandy or our special favorite—Patrón® Tequila XO Café. Meringues tend to get soft in humidity, so eat em' up!

Joy's Tips & Tricks

Olive Oil

RASPBERRY

This thick, rich, perfectly balanced Balsamic Vinegar, bursts with the natural flavor of fresh, ripe raspberries.

Both sweet and tart, its perfect tossed with mixed salad greens and a little feta cheese. Also enjoy paired with one of our flavored oils or as a marinade or glaze for pork or chicken.

Mix with Walnut or Almond oil, Meyer Lemon or Garlic Extra Virgin Olive Oil

DID YOU KNOW

Olive oil has many health benefits and other uses besides being a cooking oil? You can start making your own health, beauty and household products right in your own kitchen! These items are natural, safe, chemical-free and best of all, cost effective!

But first, let us show you some time-honored dessert recipes and their healthier counterparts using olive oil!

Then, starting on page 68 we get creative, so don't put those ingredients away just yet! Judy will show you how to make her unique household products using most of the same ingredients as Joy's favorite traditional and tasty recipes.

Brownies

Has this ever happened to you? You are just about finished mixing a batch of brownies and just when you reach for the vegetable oil: "OMG...there isn't any left, now what? Can I use olive oil?" Yes you can! Adding olive oil to your brownies in place of vegetable oil will work just fine. A mild light olive oil has a mellow flavor and will make a more dense, fudgy brownie. It is delicious, and I love that I can make a small, but healthy change to this old time classic.

OLIVE OIL & COCOA BROWNIES

3	large eggs	1½	cups unbleached flour
1½	cups sugar	½	cup cocoa powder
½	cup extra virgin olive oil	1	teaspoon kosher salt
2	teaspoons pure vanilla extract	½	cup cacao nibs (optional)

Pre-heat oven to 350°F. Coat an 8-inch square baking dish with olive oil. Cut a piece of parchment to fit just the bottom of the dish and oil that too.

Beat the eggs in a heavy duty mixer for a minute. Increase speed to medium-high while adding the sugar ½ cup at a time. Beat until the eggs are pale, thick and creamy. Decrease mixer speed and slowly add the oil in a thin stream, as if you were making an emulsion-like mayonnaise. Add the vanilla extract.

Sift together the flour, cocoa and salt into a bowl. Stir into the egg mixture until incorporated, scraping down the bowl as needed. Pour the batter into the prepared baking dish and sprinkle with the cacao nibs over the top (if using).

Bake: 25-30 minutes, or until a toothpick inserted into the center of the brownies emerges with some moist crumbs. Cool the pan completely on a rack before cutting into serving pieces

Add your favorite nuts for crunch and a protein boost!!

Judy's Tips & Tricks

Brownies

THE JOY

There is nothing better than a warm brownie enjoyed by a roaring fire in the winter, or with a dollop of creamy, cold ice cream in the summer. Brownies are so versatile and a "go to" recipe for many. You can add almost anything to the batter: nuts, chips, even chopped cookies and pretzels. Frost and sprinkle with any thing you like! You can even change the shape for a more creative presentation and a smidge more elegant!

MY FAVORITE BROWNIE RECIPE

½ cup butter or margarine	1 teaspoon vanilla extract
⅓ cup premium cocoa	½ cup all-purpose flour
1 cup granulated sugar	1/4 teaspoon salt
2 eggs	1/2 cup nuts, chopped

Preheat oven to 350°F. Grease one 8-inch square baking pan.

In a medium saucepan melt the butter over low heat (or melt in microwave in a one-quart container).

Remove the melted butter from heat, add the cocoa, and stir until well-blended. Add the sugar and mix well. Add the eggs, one at a time, beating well after each addition. Stir in the vanilla, flour and salt. DO NOT OVERBEAT. Fold in the nuts.

Spread in prepared pan and bake: 25-30 minutes, or until wooden toothpick tests done.

On the second day, cut a piece and hide in a napkin in your hand. Take a bite and wave to kids as the school bus pulls away!

Joy's Tips & Tricks

Coffee Cake

THE JUDY

There are several reasons I love substituting olive oil for butter, or shortening, when I bake. First, it is always the correct temperature. Most recipes call for room temperature butter, and who has room temperature butter readily available? Second, by cutting the saturated fat and cholesterol, I feel less guilty about eating a piece (or two)!

This cake has a moist texture, and a sweet, yet pleasingly, tart bite from the lemon. Most of my days begin with this delicious cake along with my morning cuppa. I hope yours will too!

OLIVE OIL CAKE COFFEE CAKE

1 cup all purpose flour	2 teaspoons vanilla extract
½ cup almond flour	½ cup extra virgin olive oil
1 cup vanilla sugar	½ cup lemon juice
½ teaspoon salt	Zest of 1 lemon
1 teaspoon baking soda	2 eggs
1 teaspoon baking powder	Powdered sugar for garnish

Pre-heat the oven to 350°F. Oil a 9-inch cake pan and line the bottom with parchment paper.

In a large bowl, combine the dry ingredients and stir until combined. Make a well in the dry ingredients and add in the wet ingredients. Beat on medium low until everything is combined. Do not over beat.

Pour the cake batter into the oiled pan. Place in the oven and bake: 45 minutes.

The cake is done once the edges have browned and pull slightly away from the sides of the pan. If testing with a toothpick, it should come out clean. Let the cake sit for a few minutes, then run a thin knife around the sides of the cake to loosen. Carefully remove the cake from pan, place on serving dish and sprinkle with powdered sugar.

For a special presentation, use a bundt pan—just make sure to oil extremely well.

 It will take a few less minutes in the oven too if you use a bundt pan! A quicker coffee cake for when you just can't wait!

DID YOU KNOW?

Most coffee cake recipes do not contain coffee as an ingredient? The very first coffee cakes were made with honey, boiled raisins, dates and nuts—making them more like the fruit cake we know today. It was baked in a single layer pan, usually square or rectangle.

Serve the
cake warm
(my preference),
or allow it to cool
then serve

Judy's Tips & Tricks

Coffee Cake

Dessert is a big deal in our family. Before every holiday, Mom calls a meeting to plan the food. She sits at the head of the table with her paper and pen (yes, I said paper and pen, she wants nothing to do with computers) and the first item on the agenda is to plan the desserts. Her coffee cake is always on the list (justifiably so, as it is the most requested item). She uses her grandmother's recipe which has been in our family for generations. We love listening to her describe our great-grandmother Nellie, beating the cake by hand with her big strong arms. This was the secret behind why her cake would always rise so high! Everyone who has tried this cake love it. Mom always said, "a batter that is delicious raw,* will be even more amazing when baked". Well, this cake is scrumptious, so put on a big pot of coffee and enjoy!

OLD FASHIONED SOUR CREAM COFFEE CAKE

2 cups all-purpose flour	½ cup butter
1 teaspoon baking powder	2 large eggs
1 teaspoon baking soda	2 teaspoons vanilla extract
¼ teaspoon salt	1 cup sour cream
1½ cups sugar	

In a medium size bowl, mix together the flour, baking powder, baking soda and salt, set aside.

In a large bowl, cream the butter and sugar. Add the eggs, one at a time, and beat after each. Add the vanilla and sour cream, mix. Add the dry ingredients and mix until combined.

Make topping (see below).

Pour cake batter into prepared pan and sprinkle with topping. Or add half of the batter, sprinkle with topping, pour rest of batter on top, sprinkle with remaining topping and bake.

One 12-cup tube pan, buttered and floured

Set a rack in the middle of the oven and preheat to 350°F. Bake for 50-60 minutes.

TOPPING

1 cup (about 4-5 ounces) roasted walnuts, coarsely chopped
¼ cup brown sugar
2 teaspoons ground cinnamon

Sprinkle the walnuts onto a cookie sheet and bake in the oven for about 10 minutes. Watch carefully, they can brown fast. Let cool then mix with the sugar and cinnamon

* Do not eat raw batter, it may contain salmonella bacteria

DID YOU KNOW?

Coffee cake was offered as a gesture of kindness to family and friends. The cake would be served at the coffee table, or on an elaborately dressed table, set with fine china. No matter how coffee cake is served, it remains one of the world's most popular, and delicious, cakes ever.

· 58 ·

Add a couple tablespoons of balsamic vinegar to the nuts when roasting to add flavor and an irresistible sweetness. For this recipe, I like to use an espresso flavored balsamic or one with spice like cinnamon.

Butter EVOO + balsamic vinegar = reduced bad fats and sugar.

Roasting the walnuts before you use them really brings out the flavor.

Joy's Tips & Tricks

Chocolate Chip Cookies

THE JUDY

After you read my recipe I know you will be saying to yourself, "Really? These cookies taste good?" They are totally my choice over the traditional! The olive oil adds a great depth of flavor and creates a chewy, yet crunchy texture. I just can't describe it, so I won't. Just make a batch and try them for yourself. They taste great, and more importantly, I don't feel guilty about eating the whole batch!

OLIVE OIL CHOCOLATE CHIP COOKIES

2 cup all-purpose flour	1 tablespoon vanilla extract
1 teaspoons salt	³/₄ cup vanilla sugar*
1 teaspoon baking soda	³/₄ cup brown sugar
¹/₄ cup extra virgin olive oil (I like to use something a bit more exotic like a blood orange flavored oil, but unflavored extra virgin olive oil works just fine!)	2 eggs
	1 or 2 tablespoons of vanilla almond milk
	1 cup chocolate chips

Preheat the oven to 375°F.

Combine the flour, baking soda, and salt in a medium bowl and set aside.

Combine the sugars, vanilla, and olive oil and beat mixture at medium speed: 2 minutes. Beat in eggs one a time. Gradually beat in the flour mixture, then add a tablespoon of milk. If the dough is a little dry, add a bit more milk (I used 1 tablespoon + 1 teaspoon). Stir in the chips.

Roll cookie dough into balls and place on a greased or lined baking sheet and bake: 10-12 minutes, until lightly golden.

DID YOU KNOW?

The chocolate chip cookie has been a favorite for decades. Some people add oatmeal, M&M's, nuts & raisins and even peanut butter to their recipe. Anything added tastes good.... how could it not?

Chocolate Chip Cookies

THE JOY

The chocolate chip cookie is definitely the all-American cookie. We see it everywhere: at every family parties, picnics, and on holiday dessert tables (it definitely makes an appearance on my sweets platter). This recipe was given to me by my friend Cheryl, almost 30 years ago; I have experimented with the recipe over the years to get it just the way my family likes it! I think I have finally found the right texture and sweetness. I know this will become a favorite of your family's too. Enjoy!

JOY'S FAVORITE CHOCOLATE CHIP COOKIES

2 cups flour	1 teaspoon baking soda
1 bar butter flavored Crisco (1 cup)	2-3 teaspoons vanilla extract
2 cups vanilla sugar*	12 ounces good quality chocolate, chopped
1 egg	1 cup nuts, any kind, optional
1 teaspoon salt	

Preheat oven to 350°F and line a cookie sheet with parchment paper.

Beat Crisco and sugar until fluffy: 3 minutes. Add the egg and vanilla extract, mix until combined.

In a separate bowl combine the dry ingredients, blend thoroughly and add to the mixer. Stir just until incorporated. Add the chunks of chocolate, and nuts (if using), mix with a spoon until combined.

Roll into a 1¹⁄₂ inch ball onto the prepared cookie sheet and bake: 19-20 minutes or until golden (oven temperatures vary). So stay close by and watch them.

So delicious when dunked into ice cold milk!

When baking any treat, it always comes out best when all the ingredients are room temperature.

DO NOT OVER MIX.

Over mixing will lend to a tough batter.

Joy's Tips & Tricks

Apple Crumble

DID YOU KNOW?

An apple crumble is fruit on the bottom and an oat streusel crumbled on top; or is that a cobbler? or is it maybe a crisp? Do you know the difference? First let's start with the what these desserts have in common—the fruit is always on the bottom and they are baked in a baking dish. Now to their differences. Crisps and crumbles both have streusel topping, however a crumble also has oats. A cobbler on the other hand, uses biscuit dropped on top of the fruit to form a crust that looks like cobble stones!

THE JUDY

Apple anything is one of my favorite choices for dessert. I love my Mother's apple pie, and my grand-mother's apple cake is to die for. First she dips the apple slices in a sugar and cinnamon mixture, and then places them on top of the batter. I remember her making this all the time when I was a child. As much as I love these recipes the way they are, I wanted to cut down on the fat and sugar to make it a healthier option for me (so I can have it more often). So here it is...baked apple with a crumble topping. For the crumble, I used almond flour, no sugar and a heart-healthy olive oil plus a few other ingredients to spice it up. This one is totally delish and so healthy too.

BAKED APPLES WITH AN OLIVE OIL CRUMBLE TOPPING

4 large apples, cored and hollowed out	½ teaspoon apple pie spice
⅔ cup flour (I used regular white)	1 teaspoon vanilla extract
⅔ cup almond meal	½ teaspoon orange extract
⅔ cup oats	½ cup extra virgin olive oil
¼ teaspoon salt	

Place all of the ingredients, except the oil(!), in the food processor and give it a whirl. Add the olive oil in a slow drizzle until the mixture clumps...now STOP! It's done. Stuff the apples.

Preheat oven to 375°F. Coat the bottom of baking dish with olive oil, and place stuffed apples in dish. Add ¼ cup water to bottom of baking pan. Bake for about 40 minutes. Spoon juices over top before serving.

P.S. I added a handful of nuts for added crunch!

Baked apples are great served as a side dish with pork or turkey.

Judy's Tips & Tricks

Apple Crumble

THE JOY

I have been baking this dessert for family and friends for a number of years now, always adding a bit more of this, or a pinch more of that. I think I finally got it just right! Somehow though, over the years, my younger sister Jackie took over baking this dish. It was our Dad's favorite, and sadly, since he passed away, Jackie stopped making it. She just couldn't...she tried once, but cried through the whole process. This year, after Judy survived her breast cancer, she can't seem to get enough apple anything. Soooooo...my baby sister will be making this recipe again for Judy. Now, if there are any tears, they will be tears of Joy and gratitude. Yayyyyy!

DADDY'S FAVORITE APPLE CRUMBLE

2½	pounds apples, your favorite variety, peeled, cored & sliced	½-1	teaspoon grated lemon rind
			a good splash of fresh lemon juice
1	cup vanilla sugar*	2	tablespoons cornstarch mixed with ¼ cup water
2	teaspoons apple pie spice		

Preheat oven to 350°F. Butter a 9x13-inch decorative baking dish, or any size (the apples will bake down so don't worry).

Place the apples in a large skillet on medium heat, sprinkle with lemon juice.

Combine the sugar, pie spice and lemon rind in a small bowl, sprinkle over the apples and toss to coat. Bring this mixture to a boil, uncovered, about 5 minutes. Add the cornstarch/water mixture and stir to blend. Pour into prepared baking dish. Set aside.

Sprinkle the crubble topping (below) over the apples. Bake: 30 minutes, or until top is golden and the apples are soft.

CRUMBLE TOPPING

¾	cup brown sugar		pinch of salt
¾	cup flour	½-1	teaspoon cinnamon
½	cup melted butter	¾	nuts *(optional)*
½-1	teaspoon vanilla extract		

Melt the butter and let it cool slightly. Add the vanilla extract.

Add butter to dry mixture and blend. Taste it! Add a bit more of whatever flavor you like.

DID YOU KNOW?

The Second World War influenced the creation of the apple crumble? In Britain during WWII, food was rationed, so there just wasn't enough ingredients going around to make an apple pie. Out of necessity, the apple crumble was invented. It took a lot less flour to make, and was less expensive too.

Using a few different varieties of apples gives a wonderful melody of flavors and textures.

Joy's Tips & Tricks

Body Scrub

DID YOU KNOW?

Making your own body scrub is easier than you think. It's certainly less expensive than buying one, or going to a spa. But more importantly, it is chemical-free, made only with natural ingredients.

Banana flesh is very hydrating and great for wrinkles as a topical treatment. It improves the texture of skin by toning it up and adds a healthy glow!

THE JUDY

I totally love this body scrub because everything in it is good for you, plus it's safe enough to eat . Could it get any better? As soon I mixed ingredients together, I was imagining myself enjoying a big delicious slice of my mother's banana bread slathered in butter. But this recipe has no calories; it goes on your body, not in.

The bananas are creamy and blend nicely with the olive oil giving the scrub a nice, luxurious feel. The sugar, sea salt and nuts add the right amount of texture for a great scrub, while the vanilla and cinnamon makes the experience just delicious!

P.S. *I added the salt last so I could eat some of the mixture. Don't tell anyone!*

BANANA NUT BREAD BODY SCRUB

2-3 bananas	⅛ cup ground walnuts *(optional)*
1 teaspoon olive oil	1 teaspoon of vanilla extract
¾ granulated sugar	½ teaspoon of cinnamon
½ cup course sea salt	

Mash the bananas with a fork in a bowl. Add the remaining ingredients. Put in an air tight container and store in the fridge for 2-3 days.

Use a plastic container. The scrub may be a little slippery, due to the olive oil, and could slip out of your hands in the bath or shower.

Banana Bread

THE JOY

These tender little cakes are super moist. The healthy flours and the coconut oil are great choices for baking any sweet treat. Topped with a drizzle of local honey, and garnished with a few periwinkle flowers; the presentation is really the top banana. Plus, they're gluten free!

BABY BANANA BUNDT CAKES

2 medium bananas, mashed	1½ teaspoons baking soda
2 tablespoons coconut oil, melted	½ teaspoon salt
1 tablespoon honey	1 teaspoon cinnamon
1 tablespoon vanilla extract	¼ cup chopped almonds *(optional)*
3 eggs	honey for drizzle
1 cup almond flour	edible flowers for garnish
½ cup coconut flour	

Preheat oven to 350°F. Grease mini bundt pans, set aside.

Mix together the bananas, coconut oil, honey, vanilla, and eggs until completely combined. Add the almond flour, coconut flour, baking soda, salt, and cinnamon stir until all the ingredients are fully incorporated.

Spoon the mixture (which should be thick) into the prepared mini bundt pans and smooth the top. Sprinkle the chopped almonds over the top. Fills about five mini bundt pans.

Bake for 20-25 minutes or until the bread is golden brown and a knife comes out clean. Let cool for 10 minutes, then invert onto a wire rack to cool completely.

Drizzle with honey and garnish with edible flowers (*if using*).

Not a fan of Coconut? Try using Almond or Walnut Oil

Joy's Tips & Tricks

DID YOU KNOW?

Olive oil alone can be used as a makeup remover (and it works beautifully), but when mixed with coconut oil, this delightful mash is now fantastic!

Coconut oil is a natural plant based oil and is great for hydration.

Olive oil is full of polyphenols which are an antioxidant, as well as anti-inflammatory. In the skin care world even the word inflammation is known to cause wrinkles!

The combination of these two ingredients glide across your skin, and break down the makeup; making it easy to remove when using a tissue or a cotton ball.

Olive Oil and Coconut Smash

THE JUDY

I use a waterproof foundation everyday, and rarely go out without it. One day, I realized I didn't recognize any of the ingredients in my makeup remover. My remover? The one my mom said was perfect for me to use at 13-years old? Oh my gosh, have I really been putting all those chemicals on my face for that long? My Mom needs to re-think this, I certainly have. I love the way this Olive and Coconut Oil Smash makeup remover is so smooth and velvety, it melts deliciously into your skin the second you put it on. I wipe it away with a tissue and cleanse as usual.

OLIVE OIL AND COCONUT SMASH MAKEUP REMOVER

- 6 parts coconut oil (6 tablespoons)
- 2 parts light olive oil (2 tablespoons)

Place both ingredients in a small bowl. Smash together with a spatula until mixed.

 This makes a great gift for a birthday girl. Especially one who just started to use face make-up. I like to store in fun shaped plastic containers for the teenagers—it could be a little slippery and drop!

For a firmer texture, keep your smash in the refrigerator, or in the cabinet for a softer mixture.

Judy's Tips & Tricks

Olive Oil Mayonnaise

THE JOY

Store-bought mayo is incredibly nasty. Aside from the questionable ingredients, those mayos are made with industrial oils—completely toxic and awful for your body.

I love this recipe for mayonnaise. The thought of giving up our favorite summer picnic salads was something we just couldn't imagine. Now we don't have to; tuna, macaroni, potato and chicken salads will live on in our homes with this clean, great-tasting mayonnaise.

This recipe uses amazingly-healthy coconut oil and real olive oil, along with fresh pastured eggs. A pastured egg is from a chicken that is allowed to roam in an open field, the way you might imagine a chicken would want to live!

A HEALTHY MAYONNAISE? YES!

- 1 whole, pastured egg
- 2 pastured egg yolks
- 1 tablespoon Dijon mustard
  Juice of 1/2 small lemon
- ½ teaspoon sea salt

- Pepper to taste
- ½ cup extra virgin olive oil.
- ½ cup coconut oil, extra-virgin or refined
  Secret ingredient:
- 1 tablespoon plain whole milk yogurt

Melt your coconut oil over a very low heat setting, just so it turns from a solid to a liquid. Do not let it get hot, or it will cook the eggs. Slowly pour the oils into your food processor/blender while is running at low speed. It is important this is done very slowly; just pouring a very thin stream. Once the oils are emulsified, add the yogurt. Yogurt gives the mayonnaise a semi-sweet and tangy flavor and helps it to stay fresh.

Pastured eggs
are available at
Whole Foods, and
other speciality
grocery stores.

Joy's Tips & Tricks

Body Butter

THE JUDY

Have you ever really looked at all the lotions you have in your bathroom? I must have ten! One for my body, one for my hands, one specifically for my feet, the list goes on and on. Like most of you, I have been slathering this stuff on for years. Really? This is ridiculous and I headed straight to my kitchen to test out some homemade recipes. I had most of the ingredients right in my home and the rest I ordered online. Within a few days, I was whipping up batches of body butter to die for, and so can you, here's how.

WHIPPED CHOCOLATE BODY BUTTER

1 cup cocoa butter	½ cup mild/light olive oil
½ cup coconut oil	1 teaspoon of chocolate extract

Using a double boiler, melt the cocoa butter and the coconut oil until it becomes liquid. Stir in the olive oil.

Chill this in the fridge, just until it begins to harden, but not completely hard. Using any mixer (hand held or standing) mix till peaks form.

Fill any container you like, and chill for an hour or so.

This makes a great gift!

If your house is warm, keep in the refrigerator; or it may go back to a liquid form. If so, no worries, just chill again and re-whip!

Judy's Tips & Tricks

Vanilla Cupcakes

THE JOY

You say, olive oil in a cupcake?" yes! People often want to substitute vegetable oil in their baking recipes with olive oil because they know that olive oil is a 'healthy' oil. It's true that olive oil is a poly-unsaturated fat, which makes it a healthy oil. Olive oil will react in the same way with most baking recipes in the same way as other vegetable oils.

OLIVE OIL VANILLA CUPCAKES

2	cups all purpose flour (or substitute gluten-free flour)
1	cup vanilla sugar*
1	teaspoon baking soda
1	teaspoon baking powder
½	teaspoon salt

2	eggs (or egg substitute)
1	cup vanilla soy milk (or any type of milk: dairy, almond, coconut)
1	tablespoon vanilla extract
3	tablespoons extra virgin olive oil
¼	teaspoon lemon juice

Pre heat oven to 350°F.

Whisk together dry ingredients in a mixing bowl. Add in the wet ingredients (starting with eggs), and beat with a hand mixer until smooth: 2 minutes.

Divide batter evenly into 12-lined muffin cups. Bake: 22-25 minutes, or until tops are lightly browned and a toothpick inserted into the center of the cupcakes comes out clean.

*Vanilla Sugar: 2 cups white sugar, 1-2 fresh vanilla beans, split in half.

VANILLA WHIPPED CREAM FROSTING

1	cup heavy cream
2	tablespoons agave

½	tablespoon coconut extract
1	tablespoon vanilla extract

Place the cream, agave and extracts in a large bowl. Whip with a mixer until stiff peaks form.
Makes about 2 cups

A stiff peak is when you lift the beaters. The peaks should stand straight up.

Joy's Tips & Tricks

Orange Dreamcicle

THE JUDY

Our father had a beautiful voice and loved to sing. He sounded a lot like the Chairman of the Board, Mr. Frank Sinatra. When he was young, he sang at all the ballrooms and night clubs in town, loving every minute of it. His mother, our Gramma, would tell us this about how he would come home with such a sore throat from singing to all the girls!! She would give him a teaspoon of olive oil and tell him to let it to trickle down the back of his throat. I can still see her smiling face as she said, "He always gave me a big kiss and said thanks Ma!"

My youngest son seems to have inherited "the voice" and often asks me for the old-fashioned family remedy. However, I've added a few delicious ingredients so he would like it better. I think you will too!

ORANGE DREAMSICLE SORE THROAT SOOTHER

1	tablespoon extra virgin olive oill		¼	teaspoon orange extract
½	teaspoon honey or agave		¼	teaspoon vanilla extract

Place all of the ingredients in a small cup, mix well. A teaspoon every once in a while does the trick!

DID YOU KNOW?
Olive oil is great for coating and soothing a sore throat that feels dry and scratchy. Just a bit is all you need for some quick relief.

Mix before using, the ingredients may tend to separate.

Judy's Tips & Tricks

Citrus Dressing

THE JOY

I love all these wonderful, but unusual, flavors for a salad. Orange and vanilla work so great together and adding honey makes it a great combination. Most people do not think of sweet when they think of salad dressings; but I like to think out of the box sometimes and shake up my traditional recipes. The scent of the citrus reminds me of summertime, warm weather and a salad my Nana would make during trips to our family cottage. I have added a few more ingredients to her original recipe and love to serve it anytime of the year.

ARUGULA, FENNEL AND ORANGES WITH A CITRUS DRIZZLE

1	large fennel bulb		4	cups fresh arugula
3	navel oranges			vinaigrette *(see below)*

Cut off the stems and feathery fronds and remove any bruised or discolored outer layers. Cut the fennel bulb in half lengthwise, removing the tough parts of the core. Next cut the bulb in half crosswise, and then into slices about a half inch thick, finally cut the slices into 1-inch pieces.

Peel the oranges and separate sections.

Place the fennel and arugula in a large serving bowl. When ready to serve, drizzle the vinaigrette over the arugula and fennel and toss gently to coat. Arrange the orange slices on top. Drizzle with as much of the remaining vinaigrette as you like and serve right away.

CITRUS VINAIGRETTE

2	teaspoons grated orange zest		2	teaspoons Dijon mustard
1/4	cup fresh orange or tangerine or clementine juice		1	shallot, finely chopped
2	tablespoons fresh lemon juice		1/2	teaspoon dried tarragon (optional)
4	tablespoons extra virgin olive oil			Salt and freshly ground pepper
1/2	teaspoon vanilla extract			

In a small bowl, whisk together the orange zest, orange juice, lemon juice, olive oil, vanilla, mustard, shallot, and tarragon (if using). Season to taste with salt and pepper. Set aside.

Peppermint

THE JUDY

When preparing for our TV cooking segments, Joy and I are on our feet constantly for three days prior to the show. One day is spent shopping for the set: getting dishes, pots, pans, and etc. One day to bring everything back, because Joy changed her mind overnight. And one day to actually bake and test the recipes. Finally, it's show day—and we wear heels! Our feet are tired, hot, sweaty, and they ache...ugh!

During all this, it helps to treat your feet with a soothing rub! I massage a few drops of this on my feet at night before bed. It feels wonderful, enjoy!

PEPPERMINT OIL FOOT RUB

15   drops of peppermint essential oil
     just slightly under 1 ounce of olive oil

Fill a one ounce dropper bottle with olive oil just under full, add peppermint drops. I used 15 peppermint oil drops, add as many as you like. Be careful though, peppermint essential oil is strong. When adding drops, I only add 5 drops add a time then shake the bottle to mix. Take a sniff, add more drops if needed.

After I massage the oil into my feet I put on a pair of nice white cotton socks to keep from ruining my sheets. (I use any color socks that are clean that day!)

This is a great gift for a girlfriend's birthday, add a soft pair of socks to go with it!

Ask your spouse or significant other to do the massage for you...it feels even better!

Judy's Tips & Tricks

Peppermint Gelato

THE JOY

There is something about ice cream, or in this case gelato, that makes everyone smile—including me. Now you know that I love to make everything homemade, and never ever take the easy way out, but just this once I am! Everyone is allowed that once or twice in their lifetime. I happen to like the gelato that is on the market these days. When I go to my favorite store, I buy their best, freshly-made vanilla. Once home, I add peppermint extract and throw in my homemade olive oil chocolate chip cookies and brownies; cut up into chunks.

PEPPERMINT ICE CREAM WITH OLIVE OIL BROWNIES AND COOKIE CHUNKS

1   pint vanilla gelato

1   teaspoon peppermint

1   olive oil chocolate chip cookie, crumbled *(see recipe on page 12)*

1   olive oil brownie, crumbled or chopped into small chunks *(see recipe on page 4)*

Soften gelato by leaving out for a bit. Fold in the crumbled cookies, brownie and peppermint. Taste and add more peppermint if you like.

Joy's Tips & Tricks

Homemade Bug Spray

THE JUDY

After a long day I like to sit out on the back porch, sip my decaf coffee and just listen to all the night air has to offer. Unfortunately, that often means mosquitos here in the north east. As I move into a healthier lifestyle, I know I can make better choices about what I put on my skin. I am going slow. It is very easy to become over whelmed with all these changes, but a homemade mosquito spray oil is definitely one change I am interested in. Making the spray was a lot easier than I thought. It's inexpensive, and I must admit, kind of fun. I loved picking out all of the essential oils used in this potion. Try it, I think you will like it.

HOMEMADE OLIVE OIL BUG SPRAY

4	ounces of distilled water
4	ounces Witch Hazel
½	teaspoon very light olive oil

25	drops clove essential oil
25	drops cinnamon essential oil

In an 8 oz spray bottle add all ingredients and shake well before each use. I used an olive oil mister

 Do not use on children. Wash hands after use.

Always do a test on yourself for minor skin irritations. Do not use on your face.

Judy's Tips & Tricks

Simmering Spice Oil

THE JOY

When I want the house to smell like the fall, and feel all warm and cozy; I make my own simmering oil and throw in a few cinnamon sticks and a small handful of cloves. I save all the last few drops (that isn't enough for a recipe) of olive oil from the bottom of the bottle in a little jar. By the time the holidays roll around I have just enough to make spice simmering oil!

It smells wonderful. Go ahead and give it a try!

CINNAMON AND CLOVE SIMMERING OIL

1/2	cup oil
2-3	cinnamon sticks
	small handful of whole cloves

Add all ingredients to your favorite simmer pot and enjoy!

Add small
pieces of orange peel,
star anise ...anything
you like!

Joy's Tips & Tricks

Sun Protection

THE JUDY

After reading up on some of the ingredients in store bought sunscreens, I decided that I should try to make my own using natural ingredients. I now need to stay out of the sun when it is at its strongest, and enjoy being under an umbrella a bit more; but I find it worth it, knowing I did not slather cancer causing chemicals all over my body.

HOMEMADE SUN PROTECTION

- 1/2 cup olive oil
- 1/4 cup beeswax
- 1/4 cup coconut oil

- 2 tablespoons of non-nano Zinc Oxide. Do not inhale, I wear a mask.
- A few drops of an essential oil. (I like lavender mixed with a bit of vanilla essential oil also!)

Add all ingredients, except the zinc oxide, in a glass jar that is at least a pint or larger. I love the mason jars you can get at the grocery store.

In a medium sauce pan, add a few inches of water and warm over medium heat. Put the glass jar in with the cover on loosely until the ingredients start to melt. Stir a few times to mix. When completely melted add the zinc oxide and stir until combined.

Take out of water carefully, may be hot and let cool. Stir a few times as it is cooling.

Store in a dry cool space.

Use a mask when working with the Zinc Oxide.

I prefer a thicker consistency, so I used a bit more beeswax..

Judy's Tips & Tricks

Orange Shortbread Cookies

THE JOY

I just love cookies, but a cookie with olive oil? Yes! I try to only make them when I'm having guests over so I don't eat all of them myself. The richness of the olive oil as opposed to butter is great in a shortbread cookie (and I was skeptical at first!). They are wonderfully crunchy with the olive oil and the sea salt is perfectly paired with the sweet cookie. Enjoy!.

ORANGE OLIVE OIL SHORTBREAD COOKIES WITH ITALIAN SEA SALT

3 cups all-purpose flour	1½ teaspoons sea salt
1½ cups confectioners' sugar	2 tablespoons fresh orange juice
1 cup extra virgin olive oil	sanding sugar for garnish

In the bowl of an electric mixer, combine the 1½ cups sugar and olive oil. Beat on low until smooth.

In a separate bowl, combine the flour and sea salt. Gradually add the flour mixture to the olive oil. Beat until combined (it will be crumbly).

Use your hands to roll the dough into a log that is 1-inch in diameter. Roll log in wax paper and refrigerate for one hour.

Preheat oven to 350°. Slice the dough and place on a cookie sheet. Bake for 12 minutes. Remove and place on rack.

Sprinkle with sanding sugar.

I used 1/2 teaspoon orange extract if you do not have orange olive oil.
Judy likes them baked a bit longer, until very golden brown...just saying.

If you can find blood oranges, use them...the taste is even better!

Joy's Tips & Tricks